Blossoming Beginnings

Navigating the Transformative Journey of Pregnancy

By

Martin A. Shelby, Dr.

Table of Contents

Chapter I

Creating the Scene

.

Taking on the Unknown

The attraction of the unknown is what started this life-changing journey. A mysterious journey, pregnancy is a careful dance between optimism and uncertainty. Expectant mothers are guided through the early echoes of their journey in this chapter, which emphasises the need of accepting the unexpected and finding comfort in the beauty of the unknown.

Getting Through the Emotional Maze

"Exploring the purpose and essence of 'Blossoming Beginnings '" explores the complex range of emotions that surround the life-changing experience of pregnancy. It threads through the complex web of emotions, from the first twinge of happiness to the subtle nuances of anticipation and fear. This chapter aims to establish an emotional connection with the you through evocative storytelling, so they may relate to it while they navigate the unknown waters of parenting.

The Orchestra of Life Playing Out

Think of this introduction as the symphonic opening movement that opens the subsequent harmonising chapters. It asks you to listen in to the beat of life as it unfolds, where each kick, whisper, and emotion is a note and song. In addition to being a book, "Blossoming Beginnings " is an invitation to participate in the great orchestration of creation, a journey that initiates the harmonious relationship between a mother and her child.

Exposing the Goal

The narrative's unfolding of the entwining themes of self-discovery, resilience, and the infinite love that accompanies the journey of pregnancy reveals the literary odyssey's aim. It's a call to accept this time's transforming potential, not just as a bodily phenomenon but also as a deep makeover of the soul. This chapter breaks through preconceived notions to reveal the layers of meaning woven throughout "Blossoming Beginnings ."

"Blossoming Beginnings "'s core

One finds a celebration of life in all its complexity when delving into the core of "Blossoming Beginnings ." This story explores the emotional, spiritual, and psychological aspects of pregnancy in addition to its purely biological aspects. The key is to understand that pregnancy is more than just a physical occurrence; it is a comprehensive, life-changing experience that is tightly linked to and deeply entwined with both mother and child
A Wisdom Tapestry

Allow the essence of "Blossoming Beginnings " to reverberate in the spaces between your thoughts as we set off on this fascinating journey through the pages that follow. Every page shows the minute intricacies of this life-changing adventure, like a brushstroke on a painting. I hope the knowledge imparted in these chapters serves as a beacon, shedding light on the unknown and providing comfort in accepting the journey's uncertainties. We will reveal the knowledge woven into the fabric that surrounds the internal flowering of life in the upcoming chapters.

Chapter II

Accepting the Seed: Inception and Initial Findings

The marvel of creation is shown in the silent dance of two souls becoming one, like a complex prelude to the magnificent symphony of life. "Embracing the Seed," this chapter, allows you to go into a thorough investigation of the profound journey from the beginning of life to the early phases of pregnancy, revealing the wonders and mysteries involved in the birth of a new existence.

Recognising the Conception Miracle

The Genetic Alchemy Dance

The amazing process of conception—a delicate merging of cells that signifies the beginning of life—lays the groundwork for every pregnancy. This part explores the fascinating dance of genetic material, going deep into the biological details. The microscopic marvels that begin the amazing adventure of pregnancy are explained to you, taking them from the exquisite moment of fertilisation to the early stages of embryonic growth.

The Genetic Symphony and Environment's Role

This section delves into the complex interactions that arise from the combination of genetic material and environmental influences. It explores the intriguing conversation between nature and nurture, shedding light on the ways in which the outside world shapes the developing life inside. Knowing the wonder of conception is looking beyond the molecule to the larger picture of the complex architecture of life.

Getting Through the Early Pregnancy Stages

The Womb Sanctuary

When the fertilised egg finds a home in the womb, the process of becoming pregnant begins. In this part, the delicate balance between growth and development is explored as expectant moms are guided through the earliest stages. you explore the events that occur during these fundamental weeks, from the creation of the embryonic framework to the emergence of small limbs. Comprehensive explanations are given of the complex processes involved in placental development, implantation, and the creation of the life-sustaining bond between mother and child.

Understanding Life's Early Signs and Symphonies

Getting through the early phases requires listening for the faint signals and internal symphonies of life. This section provides a thorough guide to identifying the physical changes, both subtle and overt, that indicate a flowering existence. Expectant moms are urged to connect with the deep knowledge of the life growing inside, from the first morning sickness whispers to the heartbeat that sounds like a soft melody.

Physical and Emotional Factors to Consider During This Important Time

Emotional Resonance and Hormonal Ballet

The process of becoming pregnant from conception to the early stages of pregnancy is not only physical but also very emotional. This section explores the hormonal dance that goes along with the first steps, looking at how hormone surges affect the emotional and physical domains. Expectant moms must carefully manage the emotional terrain, which ranges from the joy of finding new life to any potential worries or uncertainties. A comprehensive understanding of the complex interactions between the mind and body is provided by integrating talks on the physical changes taking place inside the body of the pregnant mother with practical techniques for emotional well-being.

Modifications to Lifestyle and Self-Care Practices

Given that early pregnancy is a holistic process, this section offers recommendations for lifestyle changes and self-care practices. Expectant moms have the ability to create an environment that is beneficial to their own health as well as the health of the growing embryo by making choices about their food and exercise regimen. It delves into the mutually beneficial relationship between mental and physical well-being, encouraging an outlook that recognises the transforming power of this pivotal time.

Taking Care of the Seed: An Appeal for Mindful Parenting

Spiritual Communion and Mindful Connection

"Embracing the Seed" invites parents to practise conscious parenting in addition to discussing the biological details. It invites you to consider conception and its early phases as a spiritual and emotional encounter in addition to a physiological reality. This episode explores the deep relationship that mindfulness and purposeful awareness can have with the seed of life. Expectant parents are encouraged to share in the spiritual significance of this life-changing experience, realising the sanctity of every moment as life's seeds sprout.

Understanding the Great Responsibilities

Pregnant parents are guided by the chapter to welcome the seed of life with mindfulness, thankfulness, and an awareness of the great responsibility that comes with fostering the fragile beginning of a new chapter. The chapter is woven together as a tapestry of information and gentle insights. The complex dance of life's unfolding is depicted as a collaboration between parents and the developing life inside, highlighting the holy responsibility to create an atmosphere that supports the developing embryo's physical, emotional, and spiritual needs.

An Introductory Note to the Innate Flower

This chapter serves as an introduction to the exciting voyage that is yet to come. It establishes the groundwork for a closer relationship with the life developing inside by painstakingly revealing the wonders of conception and the early phases of pregnancy. The journey unfolds as we turn the pages, with the seed of life growing into a vivid blossom and promising a story that goes beyond the biological to encompass the emotional, spiritual, and transforming nature of pregnancy. you are invited to immerse themselves in the rich tapestry of life's genesis as the delicate nuances of its early phases are portrayed with complex strokes.

Chapter III

Taking Care of the Bloom: Mental and Physical Health

The chapter "Nurturing the Bloom" presents a sensitive investigation of the holistic well-being of pregnant moms inside the tender embrace of approaching motherhood. This chapter sheds light on the significance of giving both physical and mental health first priority and cultivating the budding life within with kindness and awareness, going beyond the physiological changes.

Making Self-Care a Priority and Keeping a Healthy Lifestyle

The Holy Ceremony of Self-Repair

This section explores the significance of self-care as the body becomes a sacred vessel with the ability to nurture new life. Expectant women receive guidance on how to carve out time for themselves during this life-changing experience. Through the use of gentle exercises and relaxation techniques, the chapter promotes a holistic approach to self-care that nurtures the mind, body, and soul.

Creating a Healthful Way of Life

This section goes beyond standard self-care routines to discuss creating a nourishing lifestyle. The story deliberately incorporates dietary recommendations, appropriate exercise regimens, and the significance of getting enough sleep. The chapter functions as a manual to assist pregnant moms in creating a lifestyle that promotes both their own health and the best possible growth and development of the inner blooming life.

Taking Care of the Emotional Aspects of Pregnancy

Motherhood's Emotional Tapestry

Each colour of the emotional tapestry that is pregnancy adds to the bright spectrum of parenting. This part explores the subtle emotional aspects of the trip, recognising the emotional terrain of the pregnant woman and its beauty as well as its hardships. you are asked to gracefully and compassionately weave their way through this emotional tapestry, which includes everything from the exuberant expectation of motherhood to possible worries and mood swings.

Interaction and Establishment

Building a strong connection with one's emotions and using efficient communication are key to navigating emotional complexities. This section of the chapter offers advice on having honest conversations with family, friends, and partners. It supports the formation of a loving environment where emotions are acknowledged, expressed, and welcomed as vital parts of the transforming journey.

Useful Advice for Sustaining Health During Gestation

Conscious Activities for Physical Health

In this section, practical advice for preserving physical well-being is highlighted. Expectant women are armed with practical advice on everything from appropriate and safe exercise regimens to posture awareness and clean sleeping practices. The chapter serves as a companion by providing helpful advice that enables women to value and take care of their evolving bodies while being aware of the particular requirements of each stage of pregnancy.

Including Relaxation Methods

The experience of pregnancy involves more than simply bodily changes—it also involves spiritual uplift. This area offers a variety of relaxation techniques that are specifically designed to offer emotional support, such as deep breathing exercises and mindfulness meditation. In order to build an atmosphere that is beneficial to both physical and mental well-being, expectant women are advised to create moments of peace within the hectic rhythms of life.

Accepting the Whole Bloom

Combination of Mental and Physical Health

The chapter develops into a synthesis of mental and physical health. A comprehensive strategy for fostering the bloom inside consists of putting self-care first, attending to emotional subtleties, and putting helpful advice into practice. The chapter helps you understand how the body and mind are intertwined and creates a setting where the soft embrace of general well-being nurtures the burgeoning life within.

An Appeal for Mindful Parenting

The last line of "Nurturing the Bloom" urges mothers to practise attentive parenting. The chapter encourages aspiring mothers to see mental health and self-care as essential aspects of being a mother, rather than as standalone pursuits. Women are empowered to take on the job of nurturers with resilience, elegance, and an unwavering devotion to the blossoming life they carry when they take care of the emotional and physical gardens that grow within them. The chapter ends with a beacon that points you towards a path of mindful motherhood: one that embraces the blooming journey with open hearts and expanded spirits, acknowledging the complex dance of physical and emotional well-being.

Chapter IV

Foundations of Attachment: Forming a Relationship with Your Developing Child

The chapter "Roots of Connection" reveals the remarkable journey of forming an early bond—a symphony of emotions, whispers, and shared energies that lay the basis for a lifetime of connection—in the delicate dance between mother and the unborn child. This chapter explores the practice and importance of developing a close relationship with the developing life inside.

Investigating Ways to Establish a Bond with the Unborn Child

The Touch Language

Within the quiet haven of the womb, touch takes on a language all
its own. The importance of physical touch is discussed in this
section, including soft massages, peaceful times spent together,
and gentle caresses. Expectant moms receive instruction in the art
of touch, which helps them develop a bond with their unborn child at
a young age. The power of tactile communication is highlighted in
this chapter, from belly rubs to perceiving small movements.

The Sounds of Interaction

With its gentle vibrations, sound builds a bridge between a mother
and her child. This section presents techniques for fostering
connection through soundscapes, such as listening to calming
music, reading aloud, or having thoughtful conversations. The
chapter advises expectant moms to create a loving soundscape for
their unborn child, which will facilitate their bonding process and
help with their sensory development.

The Importance of Early Attachment for Mother and Child

Emotional Coherence

Early bonding is an emotional synchrony that weaves a mother's and child's hearts together, beyond only a physical relationship. This section of the chapter acknowledges the mutual nature of a connection while examining the emotional aspects of bonding. Expectant moms are encouraged to examine their feelings in order to create a loving, peaceful, and positive atmosphere that connects with their inner, developing consciousness.

The Basis of Safe Attachment

The importance of early bonding is revealed as the cornerstone of solid attachment throughout the chapter. The psychological advantages of early bonding are examined, with a focus on how important it is for the newborn to feel safe and trusted. Expectant women can lay a stable foundation that lasts through infancy and beyond by developing emotional attunement.

Building Sense of Community with Mindfulness

Being Aware During the Trip

The application of mindfulness as a technique to strengthen the relationship is discussed in this section. Expectant mothers receive guidance during periods of mindful present, which involve tuning in to the feelings, motions, and experiences that come with being pregnant. In order to establish a relationship that goes beyond the material and explores the spiritual aspects of parenting, the chapter promotes a thoughtful examination of the journey.

Imagination and Visual Links

Beyond the material, imagination bonding and visual linkages are investigated. In this section of the chapter, pregnant moms are encouraged to visualise their unborn child in their minds. The chapter gives women encouragement to develop a sense of familiarity and recognition with the developing life within, whether through ultrasound images, creative depictions, or personal visualisations.

Creating Traditions and Memories

Honouring Significant Occasions

The value of forming traditions and memories becomes clear as the chapter progresses. Expectant women are encouraged to create a tapestry of memories that will become treasured threads in the fabric of the mother-child bond, from marking significant occasions to documenting milestones. The chapter offers doable advice on distilling the journey's essence and creating a database of common experiences.

Establishing Rituals of Attachment

The bond between a mother and her child is anchored by rituals. This section helps new mothers establish little, important routines, like a bedtime ballad, a quiet time spent together, or a symbolic action. The chapter focuses on how rituals might help create a feeling of continuity and connectedness throughout the changing phases of pregnancy.

A Weave of Love and Attachment

Considering the Trip

Expectant moms are encouraged to consider the process of developing a link with their developing child as the chapter comes to a close. The importance of these early relationships is described as a love tapestry, a mosaic of touch, sound, emotion, and awareness that establishes the groundwork for a lifetime of experiences that are shared. Carefully tended to during pregnancy, the foundations of connection grow into the enduring threads that weave the complex tapestry of motherhood. This chapter serves as a witness to the life-changing potential of early bonding and encourages aspiring moms to welcome the journey of connection with open hearts and a deep understanding of the enduring bond they are forging.

Chapter V: Managing the Difficulties of Pregnancy through Seasons of Change

The fifth chapter, "Seasons of Change," is a moving examination of the many difficulties that come with being pregnant in the parenthood tapestry. Every stage of this transformation is like a different season, complete with its own set of struggles and victories. This chapter explores the changing seasons of change that pregnant moms experience on an emotional, physical, and psychological level.

Accepting the Physical Shifts

The Body in Bloom

The body experiences a symphony of changes as the pregnancy goes on; some are obvious, some are subtle, but all bear witness to the amazing process of generating life. This section walks expectant moms through the physical changes, covering popular ones like weight growth, changes in skin tone, and postural modifications. The chapter fosters an attitude of acceptance and positivity towards the changes that occur naturally in the body and provides insights into this process. It also inspires amazement at the amazing vessel that houses the developing life within.

Getting Around Pains and Illnesses

The chapter recognises the discomforts and illnesses that may occur throughout the physical changes. From morning sickness to back discomfort, pregnant women are offered with practical ideas and coping tactics. This part is a helpful companion, providing advice on how to manage everyday discomforts and deal with physical obstacles with fortitude and compassion.

The Emotional Excursion

Hormones and Flux of Emotion

Hormonal variations create a trip that is akin to an emotional rollercoaster during pregnancy. This section delves into the subtle emotional aspects that coincide with every trimester. From the highs of delight and anticipation to the lows of anxiety and mood swings, pregnant mothers are helped through understanding the emotional flux and enjoying the entire gamut of sensations that characterise this transforming phase.

Handling Fears and Anxiety

Anxieties and concerns that may develop also alter with the seasons. This section of the chapter offers a sympathetic examination of typical pregnancy-related concerns, fears, and anxieties. Techniques for recognising and resolving these issues, building emotional resilience, and establishing a safe environment for candid discussion of worries and fears are provided to you.

Developing Bonds in the Face of Change

Effect on Relationships with Partners

Pregnancy's shifting seasons unavoidably have an impact on relationships. This section looks at how it affects marital interactions and provides advice on how to keep lines of communication open, develop empathy, and work through the changing emotional terrain as a couple. It highlights how crucial it is for couples to have mutual understanding and support as they navigate the special difficulties and delights of pregnancy.

Social Dynamics and the Family

The chapter examines the impact of pregnancy on family and social dynamics in addition to partner relationships. Expectant moms receive guidance on how to set healthy boundaries, communicate with family members, and manage expectations all in the name of their own wellbeing. The chapter empowers women to build a network of support during this transformative season by acting as a resource for navigating the complexity of social relationships.

Getting Ready to Be a Parent

Waiting for It to Arrive

This part explores the anticipatory stage of preparing for parenthood as the seasons advance towards the impending advent of a new life. A number of useful options are examined, including making a birth plan, gathering baby necessities, and enrolling in childbirth education programmes. It is advised that expectant mothers seize this time of year to grow, get ready, and look forward to the moments that will change their lives.

Juggling Dreams with Actualities

As the seasons of transition culminate in the impending birth, the chapter offers ideas into striking a balance between expectations and realities. Expectant moms are encouraged in contemplating the changing path, accepting the transience of every season, and developing an attitude that embraces the unknowns of motherhood with open arms.

"Seasons of Change" encourages prospective moms to see the difficulties they face throughout pregnancy as dynamic seasons that all add to the life-changing experience of becoming a mother. you are equipped with the resilience, grace, and understanding of the ever-changing beauty found in the seasons of change to navigate the physical changes, embrace the emotional fluctuations, nurture relationships, and get ready for the upcoming parenthood season. As pregnant moms accept the joys, trials, and inherent uncertainties of the seasons that define the remarkable journey of pregnancy, this chapter serves as a guide, providing comfort and insight.

Chapter VI: Accepting the Physical Changes and Blossoming Beauty

The sixth chapter of the pregnancy journey, "Blossoming Beauty," presents a celebration of the amazing bodily changes that coincide with the conception of a child. This chapter offers advice to expectant moms on how to modify their mindset so that they see the changes as a celebration of the beauty, power, and vitality that come with bearing a child rather than as obstacles to overcome.

Honouring the Changing Physical Form

Honouring Strength

As the body experiences dynamic changes, this area enables pregnant women to celebrate the evolving physical form. The chapter examines the natural beauty in the evolving body, from the smooth curve of a growing belly to the light that comes from within. In the midst of the transformational process, it promotes a change towards self-love and appreciation and cultivates a good body image.

Mother Brilliance

Pregnancy has its own beauty that goes beyond physical changes to include a glowing motherhood. This episode delves into the science of the radiant skin and increased energy that frequently accompany pregnant women. Through accepting and honouring this inherent brightness, women are inspired to acknowledge the distinct beauty that emerges throughout this blossoming season.

Encouragement of Positive Body Image and Self-Acceptance

Redefining Beauty Parameters

This section helps expectant women to alter their definition of beauty in a culture where external appearance standards are often the driving force. The chapter encourages women to value the fortitude and resiliency their bodies have shown throughout pregnancy by promoting a body-positive society. The chapter enables pregnant moms to accept their own attractiveness by reorienting the attention from society expectations to self-acceptance.

The Magnificent Human Form

The ability of the human body to generate and sustain life is truly amazing. This section of the chapter explores the astounding features of the physiological changes, including the marvel of foetal growth, the intricate workings of the cardiovascular system, and the skin's ability to adapt. Expectant moms are guided towards a greater appreciation for the complex functions of their bodies by realising the miraculous nature of these changes.

Mental Health During Physical Shifts

Bringing Body and Mind Together

Expectant mothers' bodily experiences are closely linked to their emotional health. This section delves into the interplay between the mind and body, stressing the value of cultivating emotional fortitude in the face of physical transformations. The chapter offers advice on how to keep the physical and emotional domains in harmonic balance by practicing mindfulness, emotional awareness, and self-compassion.

Developing Emotional Hardiness

As the body develops, emotional fortitude becomes an advantageous quality. This section of the chapter offers helpful techniques for managing mood swings, dealing with everyday issues, and developing an outlook that fosters emotional health. Expectant moms can handle the changing journey with fortitude and adaptation by acknowledging and processing their feelings.

Chapter VII: Mastering the Art of Preparation: Making Parenting Plans

The seventh chapter in the mosaic of motherhood, "The Art of Preparation," serves as a helpful manual for expectant parents getting ready to welcome a new life into their home. This chapter offers guidance on preparing for the arrival of the much-awaited child by navigating the areas of logistics, planning, and emotional preparedness.

Reasonable Arrival Preparations

Putting the Nest Together

This part explores the practical aspects of being ready for parenthood, such as furnishing the newborn with a loving environment. Expectant parents receive guidance on things like nursery setup, newborn needs, and creating a safe and comfortable home environment. The chapter equips parents to create a foundation that meets the practical needs of an expanding family by taking care of the logistical aspects.

Budgeting and Financial Planning

As becoming a parent draws near, money becomes more important. This section offers guidance on how to budget and plan financially for the impending changes. Expectant parents are prepared with useful tactics for managing the financial terrain of parenthood, from comprehending the costs related to birthing to making plans for continuing expenses.

Establishing a Nurturing and Supportive Environment

Putting Support Systems in Place

Being a parent is a group endeavour, so building a strong support network is crucial. This section of the chapter delves into the significance of creating a support system that includes friends, family, and medical experts. It is advised for expectant parents to express their concerns, ask for help, and build a community that promotes a sense of shared care and responsibility.

Getting Ready Emotionally for Parenthood

Emotional readiness is just as important as practical preparation. This part walks pregnant parents through self-reflection, philosophical conversations about parenting, and techniques for emotional preparedness. The chapter helps couples align their expectations and provide the groundwork for emotional readiness for the life-changing experience of parenthood by encouraging honest conversation.

Parenting Theories and Making Decisions

Examining Parenting Approaches

As the chapter unfolds, numerous parenting approaches and beliefs are addressed. Expectant parents are encouraged to consider their parenting preferences, values, and beliefs. Couples can make decisions for their child's upbringing that are in line with their own family dynamics and goals by being aware of the many parenting philosophies.

Making Decisions as a Group

Being a parent is a team effort, thus making decisions as a team effectively becomes crucial. This section of the chapter offers advice on how to handle cooperative decision-making, settle disputes, and promote a harmonious parenting style. Expectant parents can tackle the joys and trials of motherhood together by fostering a sense of togetherness and shared responsibility.

Getting Ready for the Unexpected

Adaptability and Flexibility

Because becoming a parent is an unpredictable adventure, flexibility becomes an invaluable quality. The significance of resilience, adaptation, and accepting the unpredictable nature of parenthood are discussed in this section. Expectant parents receive guidance on developing a mindset that embraces change, manages uncertainty, and takes an adventurous attitude to the ever-evolving journey.

Self-Care in the Face of Parental Obligations

The importance of self-care in the middle of parenting obligations is underlined as the chapter comes to a close. It is advised that expectant parents put their health first, promoting a healthy balance between providing care and taking care of themselves. Couples who understand the value of self-care can enter parenting with resilience, vibrancy, and a shared commitment to their own and their developing family's well-being.

Expectant parents can use "The Art of Preparation" as a roadmap to help them navigate the logistical, emotional, and practical aspects of preparing for parenting. This chapter gives couples the tools they need to face the impending arrival of their child with confidence, readiness, and excitement for the life-changing experience that lies ahead by covering both the material and intangible aspects.

Chapter VIII

Accepting the Unknown: Getting Through the Last Trimester

The eighth chapter, "Embracing the Unknown," emerges as a roadmap for the adventure of pregnancy as it moves forward, providing guidance through the final trimester, which is characterised by a peak of expectation, careful planning, and a distinct fusion of excitement and uncertainty. This chapter offers profound insights into the physical, emotional, and practical aspects as expectant parents stand on the verge of welcoming their little one. It acts as a compass, guiding you through the complex terrain of the final stretch of the pregnant experience.

Milestones and Physical Changes

The Journey's Final Chapter

The body transforms in a symphony throughout the last trimester, indicating the impending birth of a new life. This section gently walks expectant moms through the bodily changes, including weight gain, feeling the movements of the foetus, and the body's complex labour preparations. The chapter promotes a deep connection with the impending moment of bringing the baby into the world by encouraging a conscious awareness of these changes.

Handling Uncomforts and Getting Ready for Work

During this phase, addressing frequent discomforts and getting ready for the complex dance of labour become the main priorities. This section carefully provides useful advice on how to handle bodily discomforts, recognise the subtle indicators of labour, and get ready both psychologically and physically for giving birth. Expectant parents are equipped to tackle this life-changing event with a sense of understanding, confidence, and readiness by navigating the unknowns associated with labour.

Bonding and an Emotional Rollercoaster

Looking Forward to Becoming Parents

The last trimester is an emotional rollercoaster of enthusiasm, expectation, and even anxiety. This section of the chapter turns into a lighthouse, guiding the reader over the emotional terrain with compassion and comprehension. It recognises the spectrum of emotions that could surface as the deadline draws near and offers practical methods for promoting emotional health. During this intensely emotional time, expectant parents are gently assisted in developing a closer relationship with both their unborn child and themselves.

Developing a Bond with the Infant

The importance of fortifying the emotional connection with the unborn child in the last trimester is highlighted in this chapter. Expectant parents are advised to explore different means of connecting with their infant, such as chatting to them or doing visualisation exercises, in order to improve their sense of closeness and connection. The bond between a parent and child that develops and grows after birth is woven together by this fundamental emotional connection.

Chapter IX: The Ultimate Conclusion: Handling Childbirth

The ninth chapter, "The Grand Finale," unfolds as a thorough guide through the life-changing experience of labour and delivery at the magnificent culmination of the prenatal journey. This chapter expertly handles the complex paths of birthing, providing profound understanding, useful advice, and resolute emotional support to expectant parents as they approach the momentous occasion of bringing their child into the world.

Comprehending the Labour Stages

Transitional, Early, and Active

The chapter begins by demystifying the stages of labour: early, active, and transition. Expectant parents receive a thorough road map outlining the physical and emotional subtleties of each stage, all while being gently guided through them. Parents who comprehend the stages of labour might feel empowered and equipped to handle the experience with courage, knowledge, and readiness.

Coping Strategies and Pain Control

It takes a flexible toolset of techniques to handle the rigours of labour. This section turns into a manual, going over different coping strategies like breathing exercises, posture, and movement. The chapter also explores the range of methods available for managing pain, providing information on both non-medical and medicinal strategies. With this all-encompassing approach, expectant parents can make decisions that are in line with their own preferences for childbirth.

A partner's assistance and role

The Guide for Birth Partners

Acknowledging the crucial function of the birth partner, the chapter explores the subtleties of providing labouring parents with support. This section serves as a guide for birth partners, offering advice on how to be there for the birthing parent through advocacy, constant emotional support, and active participation in the birthing process. Crucial components that foster a supportive environment during the life-changing experience of labour and delivery are effective communication and teamwork.

Building a Helpful Birth Team

The chapter delves into the idea of a supportive and coherent delivery team, going beyond the birth partner. Expectant parents are carefully guided through the process of selecting a team that is in line with their preferences for childbirth, from healthcare specialists to doulas. In order to ensure a peaceful and encouraging environment, the chapter stresses the significance of encouraging excellent communication and collaboration among the birth team members.

Greetings on the New Arrival

The Wonder of Life

This part turns into a celebration as the delivery process progresses, paying homage to the wonder of childbirth. Expectant parents receive gentle guidance during the last stages of labour, the actual delivery procedure, and the momentous occasion of the baby's arrival into the world. The chapter exhorts parents to cherish these fleeting moments in order to develop a deep sense of delight, amazement, and attachment to their newborn.

The Infant's First Moments

With insights into the early moments with the infant, the narrative comes to a close. Expectant parents are provided with helpful suggestions for their newborn's early interactions, ranging from immediate postpartum care to breastfeeding and bonding. By savouring these early times, parents create the groundwork for a caring and affectionate bond with their child that will grow throughout the course of parenthood.

Chapter X

The Postpartum Era: A Fresh Start

The tenth chapter, "A New Beginning," opens in the gentle wake of childbirth and serves as a kind guide through the postpartum phase, which is characterised by recuperation, acclimatisation, and the significant shift into parenthood. This chapter offers steadfast support and insightful guidance for expectant parents during this fragile and transforming period, while also addressing the physical, emotional, and practical aspects of the postpartum journey.

Physical Healing and Self-Surveillance

Getting Around the Postpartum Bosom

This section carefully discusses the bodily changes that are typical of the postpartum period when the body starts the healing process. Expectant mothers receive gentle guidance on postpartum healing, covering issues like postpartum haemorrhage, uterine involution, and perineal care. In order to create a sense of grace and acceptance as the body progressively adjusts to its post-birth state, the chapter advocates for a gentle and compassionate approach to self-care.

Exercise and Nutrition after Giving Birth

Incorporating postpartum exercise and nutrition into daily routines is part of physical healing. This section turns into a thorough manual, including advice on safe, progressive exercise regimens that aid in healing as well as dietary suggestions that enhance general wellbeing in the postpartum time. New parents who prioritise their physical health are better equipped to handle the rigours of parenthood with resilience and vibrancy.

Mental Health and Emotional Welfare

The Emotional Terrain of Motherhood

The postpartum phase is characterised emotionally by adjustment, delight, and occasionally difficulties. This section of the chapter develops into a sympathetic guide, skillfully negotiating the emotional terrain of fatherhood. It recognises the many peaks and valleys that could occur and offers practical methods for promoting emotional health. In this highly intense and transforming period, expectant parents are gently encouraged towards building a deeper connection with their newborn and with one other.

Identifying Mood Disorders Following Childbirth

The chapter gently brings attention to postpartum mood disorders by providing guidance on how to identify the telltale signs and symptoms of illnesses including anxiety and depression. It is advised that expectant parents place a high priority on their mental health, seek professional help when necessary, and establish a nurturing atmosphere that promotes the emotional health of both the spouse and the delivering parent.

The path to motherhood is a complex one, and "A New Beginning" serves as an insightful roadmap across the complex terrain of the postpartum phase. This chapter equips couples to face this transitional moment with resilience, compassion, and a deep feeling of enthusiasm for the new chapter that lies ahead of them by addressing both the concrete and intangible factors.

Building Family Bonds: Managing Early Parenthood is covered in Chapter XI.

The eleventh chapter, "Building Family Bonds," serves as a guide through the early days of parenting, a time characterised by deep connection, adaptations, and the development of the family unit, as the journey into parenthood continues. This chapter explores the relational, practical, emotional, and practical aspects of early parenthood, providing new parents with advice and insights as they begin this life-changing and frequently thrilling chapter.

Developing the Parent-Child Bond

Early Communication and Attachment

This part turns into a gentle manual for fostering the parent-child bond in the early stages of motherhood. In order to develop a strong bond with their newborn, new parents are urged to explore early interactions, such as skin-to-skin contact and responsive parenting. The chapter offers guidance on interpreting the baby's indications and needs in order to build a relationship that serves as the cornerstone of a stable connection.

Time Spent Together and Customs

The chapter celebrates the relevance of shared moments and rituals in developing family relationships. New parents are given guidance on how to create significant rituals and simple routines that will build the bonds within the family. These moments—be it sharing meals, cuddling in the morning, or reading bedtime stories—become the foundation of a supportive family setting.

Managing Sleep Deprivation and Changes

Overcoming Sleep Issues

The early days of parenthood are frequently accompanied with the realities of sleep deprivation. This section provides helpful advice on how to deal with sleep issues, help the baby develop appropriate sleep habits, and deal with any resulting exhaustion. In order to build resilience and adaptability in the face of changing sleep patterns, the chapter highlights the significance of self-care for both parents.

Getting Used to Being a Parent

The chapter serves as a guide for adjusting to early parenthood's adjustments. Find balance and support: new parents are helped through the process of adjusting to a new daily routine, which includes changes in roles and responsibilities. In order to help couples traverse the changing terrain of motherhood together, the chapter promotes open communication and teamwork.

Developing Parenting Values and Philosophies

Syncing Up Parenting Approaches

New parents are encouraged to examine and match their parenting philosophies and styles as the journey progresses. This section of the chapter explores how building a foundation of parenting beliefs requires open communication, mutual respect, and shared decision-making. Couples can present a united front while navigating the benefits and difficulties of early motherhood by adopting a collaborative approach.

promoting both individual and group well-being

Some tips for promoting both individual and group well-being are included in the chapter's conclusion. New parents are urged to give their physical and mental well-being top priority since they understand the value of self-care and community support. This chapter offers a guide for creating a positive and healthy family dynamic, whether that means finding time for alone, asking for help from a support system, or just spending time together.

Chapter XII

Enjoying Significant Occasions: Handling the Initial Year

The twelfth chapter, "Savouring Milestones," weaves a heartfelt narrative through the first year of a baby's life, a time of dynamic development, joyful milestones, and the subtle dance of parenthood. This chapter provides new parents with guidance and support as they cherish the priceless moments of their child's early life by illuminating the emotional, cognitive, and physical milestones of the baby's first year.

Honouring Developmental Achievers

Achievements in Motor and Cognitive Skills

The baby's developmental milestones, from the first smiles to the first hesitant steps, are celebrated in this section. New parents receive guidance on comprehending the developmental milestones related to motor and cognitive skills during the first year of life. The chapter highlights how crucial it is to create a loving atmosphere for babies that encourages curiosity and discovery, setting the groundwork for their lifetime learning process.

Social and Linguistic Development

This section of the chapter examines language and social development as the newborn starts to express themselves. It is recommended that new parents participate in interactive activities, enhance language development by creating a supportive environment and using gestures and noises to communicate. From the baby's early babble to the appearance of social grins, the chapter serves as a guide through the baby's changing social interactions.

Developing Emotional Hardiness

Emotional Connection and Parental Bonding

The importance of parental bonding and emotional connection throughout the first year of life is highlighted in this chapter. The development of a stable attachment, recognising the baby's emotional signs, and reacting sensitively are all taught to new parents. The chapter turns into a manual for building a foundation of security and trust by fostering the emotional resilience of the parents and the infant.

Managing Parental Difficulties

This section provides help for new parents in negotiating the emotional terrain of early parenthood, acknowledging the problems that may occur. This chapter offers some insights on coping skills, self-care techniques, and getting help when you need it, whether you're experiencing self-doubt or restless nights. Through accepting the ups and downs of parenthood, newlyweds can overcome obstacles with poise and fortitude.

Establishing Routines and Introducing Solids

Making the Switch to Solid Foods

The introduction of solids is covered in this section of the chapter as the baby's nutritional demands change. We offer helpful advice to new parents on how to manage this change, choose foods that are age-appropriate, and cultivate a healthy connection with food. The chapter stresses how crucial it is to view this milestone as a chance for inquiry and shared experiences.

Creating Daily Schedules

A section on creating daily routines for the family and the infant closes the chapter. New parents are urged to establish a sense of comfort and regularity via everything from playing rituals to sleep regimens. This chapter offers guidance on striking a balance between order and flexibility so that the family can create a loving and peaceful atmosphere while navigating the exciting first year of the infant.

"Savouring Milestones" provides new parents with assistance as they manage the complexities of early parenthood, serving as a testament to the delightful and transformational journey of the baby's first year. Through the establishment of healthy routines, emotional resilience building, and milestone celebration, this chapter grows to be a treasured companion in preserving the priceless moments of the baby's early life.

The book "Blossoming Beginnings : Navigating the Transformative Journey of Pregnancy" concludes with a chapter that describes the end of a deep odyssey that has been woven through conception, pregnancy, labour, early motherhood, and the milestones of the first year of life of the child. In addition to being a reflection, this last chapter extends an invitation to you to take a moment to appreciate the depth of their experiences and to welcome the continuous development of their parenting narrative.

Considering the Trip

An Upholstery of Changes

This book has weaved a tapestry of transformations, as we realise when we consider the previous chapters. Every aspect of the parenting experience, from the delicate moments of conception to the dramatic conclusion of labour and the everyday routines of early parenthood, has been a brushstroke added to the masterwork. This book sought to provide light on the relational, emotional, and spiritual aspects of the transformative journey into parenthood in addition to imparting knowledge.

Blooming Within: An Exposure to a Metaphor

The metaphor of "Blossoming Beginnings ," which stands for the deep development, grace, and resiliency that define the experience of becoming pregnant and a parent, has led us through the story. As a blossom opens up to reveal layers of complex beauty, so too does the process of bringing a new life into the world change and evolve. It is a celebration of the inner fortitude, the altruistic nature, and the developing love that characterise fatherhood.

Accepting the Continued Adventure

An Appeal for Further Development

With curiosity, resiliency, and an open heart, this conclusion issues an invitation to the you to embrace the ongoing journey that is parenthood. Parenting is a never-ending process of learning, growth, and discovery rather than a goal. The book's chapters have set the stage for you to move forward, understanding that every day brings fresh chances for happiness, connection, and strengthening family ties.

A Reminder of Fortitude and Adaptability

This book's closing remarks serve as a gentle reminder of the resiliency and strength that each and every parent possesses. Every reader is an exemplar of their own ability to love, adapt, and nurture life, from the trials of conception to the uncertainty of early motherhood. May these words serve as a source of motivation, support, and affirmation for each reader on their incredible journey forward as they go.

Final Thoughts

"Blossoming Beginnings " is a companion for the life-changing experience of becoming a parent, not just a book. May the knowledge, understanding, and kindness imparted in these chapters linger with you when they flip the last page. May the inner spirit of blooming never fade, guiding every parent on the holy and lovely path of raising a child, building a family, and relishing the constantly changing turning points of motherhood.

With loving wishes for the continuous growth of love, joy, and resilience within the fabric of your unique motherhood path.